T0146558

The Scoop on Poop

How to Make a Perfect Poo

ANNE FERGUSON BM

BALBOA.
PRESS

A DIVISION OF HAY HOUSE

Balboa Press books may be ordered through booksellers or by contacting:

Balboa Press
A Division of Hay House
1663 Liberty Drive
Bloomington, IN 47403
www.balboapress.com
1 (877) 407-4847

Print information available on the last page.

ISBN: 978-1-5043-4445-6 (sc)
ISBN: 978-1-5043-4446-3 (e)

Library of Congress Control Number: 2015918576

Balboa Press rev. date: 11/25/2015

Acknowledgements

To my mom Mrs. Ruth Ferguson & Dr. Michelle Salga for their edits, to my husband for making it possible and to all those clients who said; "You should write a book". I'm the luckiest person in the world.

Table of Contents

Introduction

About fifteen years ago, I got very ill. Although the tipping point for my illness was an injury, the big problem was an inherent failure on my part to look after my true health. One of the many ways this failure demonstrated itself in my body was through Irritable Bowel Syndrome.

Then I finally got a clue and realized that I was responsible for the condition I was in. I had to find my own way back to health. I did so through education, nutritional modification, behavior modification and colonics. It worked. When I was finally well enough to return to work, I turned this new found passion into a career and became a Colon Hydro-therapist. Elemental Therapies, a wellness centre that uses the basic elements like water and heat to heal, followed.

I love helping other people find their way to health and it is my deepest wish that the following pages help you make a perfect poo.

"www.thescooponpoop.ca"

Why Do I Care?

Have you noticed the correlation between how easy, smooth, and satisfying a bowel movement is and how well you feel?

Poo Health reflects True Health.

The title of this book is, "The Scoop on Poop; How to Make a Perfect Poo." The question you might ask yourself is, "Why do I care?"

Our digestive system is such a huge part of our health and the way that our body eliminates waste tells us how well our body is doing.

Why do we look? That's right, why do we turn around and look at what's nestled safely in the bowl?

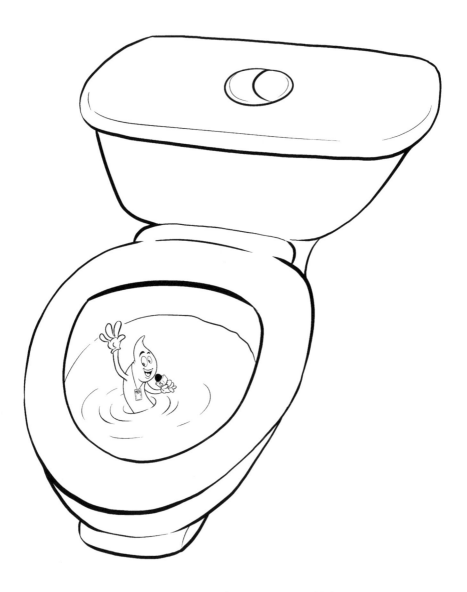

How did I know that we look? We all look. We look, because we know at a gut level (I'm talking about instinct, about unconscious awareness), that our **poo health reflects true health.**

"www.thescooponpoop.ca"

How do you feel when you have a bowel movement? Have you noticed the correlation between how easy, smooth, and satisfying a bowel movement is and how well we physically feel?

Why do we feel so crappy when our crap is crappy?

We Literally Feel Like Crap

When we have a perfect poo we feel, energetic, finished, clean. When we don't we don't.

When we feel badly after a poo it is because we had a crappy crap. If we feel good it is because we had a perfect poo.

Have you ever had a perfect Poo? One of those poos that make you feel like you can jump up and take over the world, the kind that is so satisfying you are like a new person afterward?

Our feelings are tuned to our Poo.

Or, have you ever had a hard Poo? One of those poos that you strain to eliminate, and wacks the water with such a splash you get a toilet water butt bath? Are you tired afterward? Is it nap time?

Our feelings are tuned to our Poo.

Why are our feelings tuned to our Poo? Why do we care?

Our Poo is our natural barometer. It is telling us about our health. Our poo tells us how things are going for us and provides us with a daily checkpoint.

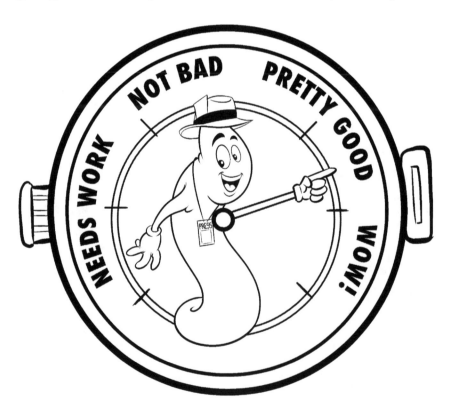

"www.thescooponpoop.ca"

When You Make a Perfect Poo You Made a Perfect You

Your body is a self building factory. Your poo is a by-product of body making. You are manufacturing you, and your poo is the waste from that manufacturing process.

It is common to consider our body a fixed substance, an unchangeable machine which runs on food and water.

The exact opposite is true. Our body is changing 24 hours a day 7 days a week 52 weeks a year, from the moment we are born, until the moment we die.

Tiny little bits of our body die every day and tiny little bits are made every day. We make ourselves.

Those tiny little bits are called cells and that is what we are made of.

We started as a single cell in our mothers' womb. By the time we were born we were a mass of trillions of cells. That mass got bigger and bigger. As it grew **cells died and fell off of us** to make room for the new fresh ones. We are a cell making factory.

But wait a minute, if cells died and fell off of us, where did they go?

The cells that are on our outside (skin, hair etc.) just drop off, the rest of them drop off and move into the lymphatic system, which then conducts them to the bladder and the bowel, so the body can eliminate these expended cells. That's right, these expended cells drop into the colon and are included as content in our poo.

When you poo, you are pooing you.

What are Good Little Cells Made of?

We need 4 ingredients to make a cell. These ingredients are the Essential Macronutrients; water, carbohydrate, fat, protein. We must consume them.

Although we don't want to get too complex, we do want to have a good understanding of the kind of things that go into making our cells because, **if it is in you, it's in your poo.**

We are what we eat. But our poo is also made up of what we eat.

Although we need many different things to build healthy cells, these ingredients can be categorized into four specific nutrients that are necessary in the cell manufacturing process. In other words, they are essential. This means we have to eat them. We must consume them. They must pass our lips.

According to popular nutrition wisdom there are only three essential macronutrients. However, water should be considered an essential macronutrient, because we must have it to build a cell. The four main ingredients that build a good cell are; water, carbohydrate, fat, and protein.

Our body is comprised of about 70 percent **water**. A readily available liquid, it serves as an excellent source of electrical conductivity, which is how our cells communicate.

Carbohydrates are a source of energy that fuels the very processes we use to build cells. They also appear inside of cells, a backup fuel source should food not be available. There are Simple

Carbohydrates and Complex Carbohydrates. For our purposes just know that the complexity of a carbohydrate is in the chew. The more complex the carbohydrate, the more chewing required.

Fat appears on the epidermis of every single cell we produce and in some cells it's the primary ingredient such as; skin cells and brain cells.

Protein is made up of amino acids. A complete total protein in an adult is considered eight different specific amino acids. These proteins are the foundation and the frame of every single cell.

Digestion Delivers
the Ingredients

The process of digestion breaks food down and delivers it to the body. The tools it uses to turn food into fuel are; Bile, Enzymes, Hydrochloric Acid, and Peristalsis Action.

The body converts those ingredients we talked about (protein, carbohydrate, fat, and water) into cells, through a very familiar process. This process is digestion. We use bile, enzymes, hydrochloric acid and peristalsis action to drive the process of digestion.

1. **Bile** is a greenish liquid that is produced by the liver and stored in the gall bladder. Its' main role is to chew up the fat.

2. **Enzymes** are released from a number of areas throughout the digestive tract, in the saliva, stomach, etc., but primarily from the pancreas. Enzymes are used to break down all the different macronutrients. There are different enzymes for each different class of macronutrient.

3. **Hydrochloric acid** is in the stomach. The primary purpose of hydrochloric acid is to break down proteins and fats. All proteins and fats are turned into a liquid substance in the stomach. Complex carbohydrates however, are not.

4. **Peristalsis action** is the behavior of the entire digestive tract. The esophagus, the duodenum, the small intestine, and the large intestine all perform a function called peristalsis. Peristalsis is a kneeding, stirring, muscular behavior, that moves food around and through the body.

From Food to Stomach

Chew, mush around, make bolus, swallow

Food follows a specific path when being digested and it goes through the same process regardless of its content. However, different macronutrients do get more attention at certain points in the digestive tract.

As soon as they enter the mouth, simple carbohydrates begin to absorb into the blood. This is because the simplest carbohydrates such as juice, white bread, mashed potatoes etc. don't require much chewing and the enzymes in the saliva are enough to cause instant absorption. Think of how, you can drink a little glass of juice and almost immediately feel the energy it provides.

Even before any food hits our mouth our body begins creating saliva, which contains enzymes that aide in the digestion of complex carbohydrates. This way, when we begin chewing, the combination of chewing and the saliva in our mouth make it easy for us to break down the food and send it through the esophagus.

Complex carbohydrates get their surface area increased through chewing. If these carbohydrates aren't chewed properly the digestive process will not be able to break them down and the nutrients are lost. If you've ever seen a red pepper or a leaf in your poo, remember, **it's all in the chew.**

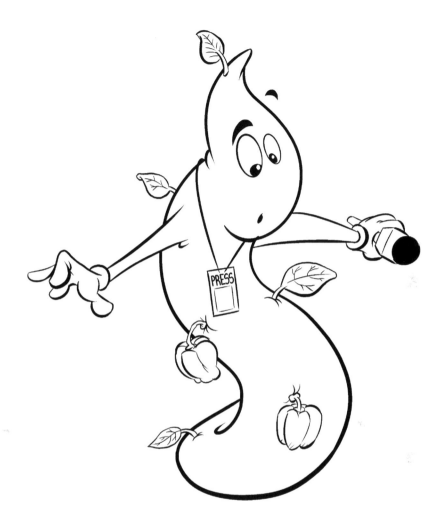

Proteins and fats get chewed up but the enzyme in saliva doesn't impact it. Chew is only important so as to get food small enough to avoid choking.

All of these items are masticated into a wad of food called **a bolus**.

The bolus is swallowed and through peristalsis and with gravity it is moved down to the lower esophageal sphincter (yes, I said sphincter), which opens up and drops the Bolus into the stomach.

From Stomach to Duodenum

Soak in acid and enzymes, then agitate

When the bolus arrives in the stomach it finds itself bathing in an acid bath. The bolus gets agitated in this bath and it breaks up into the hydrochloric acid. The acid starts to breakdown the proteins and fats that are now soaking in it. After 2-8 hours, depending on what amino acids or fat molecules were populating the bolus, the proteins and fats will have liquefied.

Stomach acid does not breakdown complex carbohydrates. You can take a raw carrot and pour hydrochloric acid on it and absolutely nothing will happen. That is why you can sometimes still see a piece of pepper or a leaf (which are complex carbohydrates) in your poop, but you never see a piece of chicken or a chunk of cheese. Thus, our complex carbohydrates leave the stomach in the same form they arrived, a chewed up enzyme soaked mess and they move through the stomach relatively quickly.

The Pyloric Valve which rests at the bottom of the stomach and opens into the duodenum regulates the pour of this chunky liquid (chyme) into the duodenum, which is the beginning of the small intestine.

To Cell or Poo? That Is the Question!

Chyme flows from duodenum, through to the rest of the small intestine, onto the large intestine, a 27 "snake.

Now this chyme moves into the small intestine. Our small intestine is astonishing and is primarily where the minerals and nutrients from the food we eat are absorbed. The small intestine can vary in size according to the individual, but can be as long as 30 ft in some people. The small intestine is made up of three parts; the duodenum, the jejunum, and the ileum.

It passes the pancreatic duct, which delivers the enzymes. There are a number of enzymes generated by the pancreas however the 3 main pancreatic enzymes are proteases, lipase, and amylase which break up proteins, fats, and carbohydrates respectively.

Then it passes the bile duct, which delivers the bile. Bile is a thick nasty substance that emulsifies the fat that passes through the duodenum.

Once past the duodenum, this new mixture of chyme will pass through the small intestine. The small intestine grabs it and, using its' peristalsis, slowly passes the chyme through its' length, kind of like an elastic band being threaded through a wasteband.

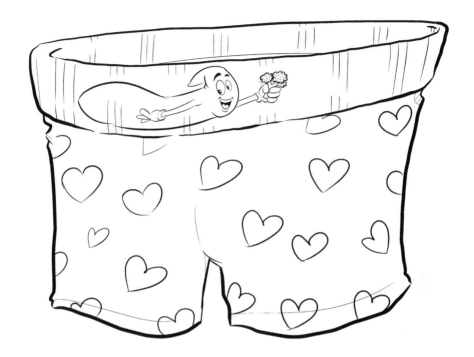

As it passes through this section of intestine, which is the width of a baby finger, the bacteria are determining what gets absorbed into the body and what moves on to the large intestine.

The ileocecal valve opens between the small intestine and large intestine and showers down the 80-90 % digested and absorbed chyme. Then the large intestine grabs it with its peristalsis action and starts to process it through its length.

This is where your poo is made by absorbing the remaining water and "packaging" your waste into fecal matter until your body is able to defecate and eliminate waste through your body.

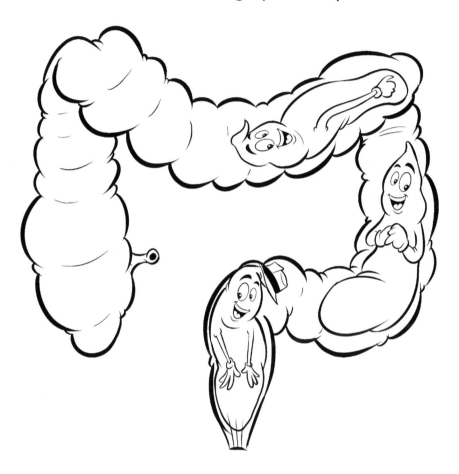

The Three Stages to Building You

Nutriating, Absorbing, Eliminating

The entire digestive process can be broken down into 3 basic stages.

1. **Nutriating:** This is my word for it anyway. Some people would call it eating, but I use nutriating to drive home what we are actually doing. This is essentially the intake portion of the process where the body intakes food, water, nutrients and vitamins. This is the most important step of the three, because without this, the other two steps cannot happen. Think of nutriating as giving your body what it needs to survive.

2. **Absorption** :This stage occurs after ingestion. So after the body has ingested food, liquid, drugs or supplements it can now extract nutrients and provide us with the calories from the source of what you ingested. This is how we get the positive benefits from the food that we eat and how we are able to benefit from healthy eating. Absorption sends nutrients into our bloodstream.

3. **Elimination**: Elimination occurs after digestion. We've eaten and we've absorbed nutrients and calories. Our body has now prepared for elimination. Our bodies take what they need from the contents of what we ingest, and then we eliminate the waste products through our bowel. If we didn't get rid of waste from our bodies it wouldn't be a pretty sight.

We are Making our Poo

We take our ingredients (whatever goes in the mouth), process those ingredients through our digestive track and output our Poo. We, through our life choices and behaviours, are making our Poo.

Remember, when you made a good poo you made a good you. Your poo tells you how well you are building your body every day. Soooo— **USE IT—** Use that time on the throne, to assess your results and correlate those results to your choices.

If I'm making my poo, and I produced the result staring back at me from the bottom of the bowl, how did I do it?

What do I do? I am a poo manufacturer and I have just produced a poo. Whether it is a Crappy Crap or a Perfect Poo now is my opportunity to figure out how I did it. When I understand how I can reproduce the process, I will know how I can make a Perfect Poo.

What if we don't take out the Garbage

Ever walked through a town on garbage strike in the dead of summer?

That's what is happening inside you.

- It's 98 Degrees

- This biodegradable product is biodegrading in you.

- Causing GAS, Bloating, Backache, Headache, Fatigue and Skin Eruptions.

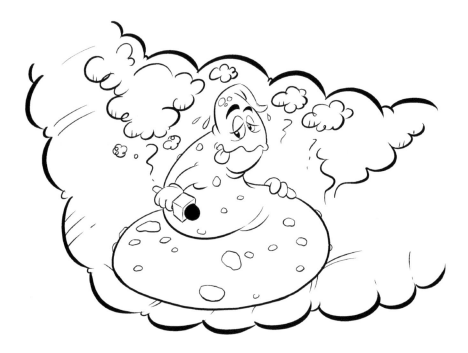

Our poo is our garbage. It's our waste. When we don't take it out, that waste just sits inside of us slowly deteriorating.

What do I mean by deteriorating? I mean this is a biodegradable product, it will degrade in this internal biological environment.

Just like garbage during a summer garbage strike, this biodegradable product, our poop, will slowly start to gas you from the inside out. That's ammonia gas which causes bloating, headache, and fatigue.

If we don't take it out, the 5 ft colon starts to fill up with poop and gas, like a balloon. It will expand, pushing along the abdominal wall and making you feel bloated. This is also pushing against the back, which is often the cause of mild to moderate backache.

Things will get worse and worse if you don't eliminate your garbage.

What's Poo To You

For perfect poo think PEERLESS poop.
For flawed feces think CRAPPY crap.

Poo is made up of more than the food you ate in the last day or so, it contains food waste, water, bile, enzymes, blood, mucous, cells and sometimes even bugs or parasites. Should you cease eating you will continue to poo,(provided the water is still coming in) because we literally poo ourselves away. The assessment of a poo must include, its texture, and ease of elimination.

When you sit on the toilet and have a bowel movement, you have the ability to see firsthand how you have been making your body. If you feel good about your poo, you will feel satisfied and proud of yourself when you get off the toilet. You will leave the bathroom with a sense of "ahhh that was good", a sigh of relief and a smile on your face. In addition to the emotional satisfaction you get, you will also notice that your poo looks peerless in the bowl. It isn't watery, hard or lumpy, and it doesn't look like rabbit pellets or a bowl of nuts. It resembles a nicely formed sausage and appears firm and well made.

A peerless poo has some oomph to it. Have you ever seen a toddler poop? They put out poops the size of an uncut deli kolbassa. It also comes to a point where you pinched off, and will not leave you with a mess that you have to wipe up with 56 sheets of toilet paper.

When pondering our poo, we can consider the following acronyms.

PEERLESS

P- Pointed

EE – Easy Elimination

R – Regular

L – Lots of it

E – Energy Burst

SS – Sausage Shaped

or

CRAPPY

C – Concrete

R – Runny

A – Atomic

P – Pencil Poop

P – Pellet Poop

Y – Yucky

"www.thescooponpoop.ca"

PEERLESS POOP

P - Pointed

- When a poop leaves the rectum it gets pinched off creating a little point.

- A tipped poo is a clean poo, it's soft and leaves a debris free anus.

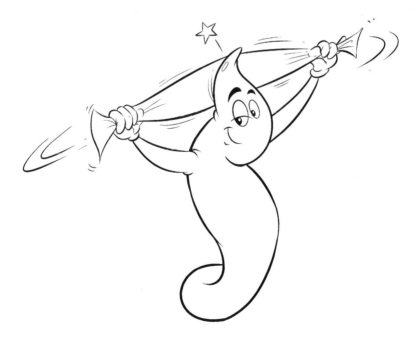

EE – Easily Eliminated

- Ease of elimination means just that, how comfortably were you able to deposit your poop in the loo?

- It should be an easy release, a gentle push and then an automatic pinch of the rectum at the end.

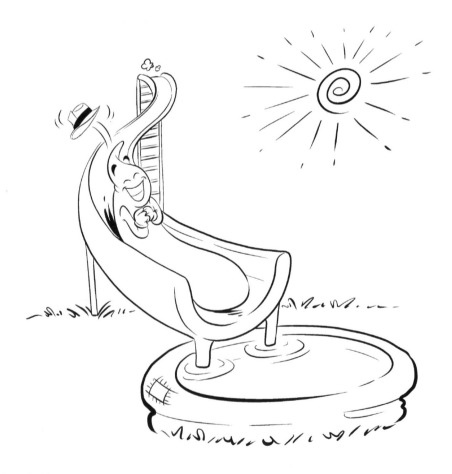

R – Regular

- The more regular a bowel movement the better.

- Once every morning after a night of sleep, and then 20 minutes or so after a meal is the ultimate frequency

- Less than once a day is not desirable.

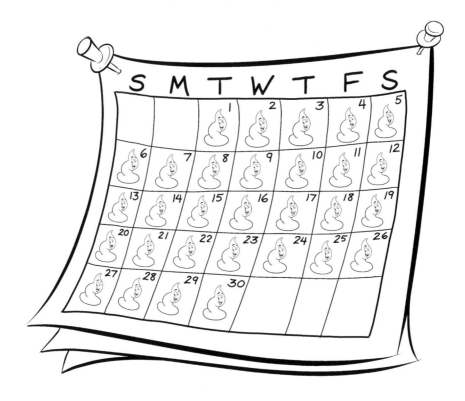

L – Lots

- It's those poos with a lot of mass that are most satisfying.

- The colon is 5 ' long and 3" in diameter and a nice active colon has lots of poop in it moving through from chyme to poo.

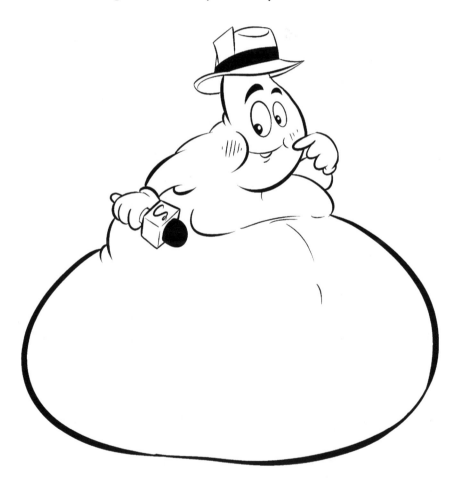

"www.thescooponpoop.ca"

E - Energy Burst

- When you've had a Perfect Poo you get a burst of energy.

- It's a sense of release and then an "OH YAHH" feeling.

- You are ready to go, start your day, take over the world.

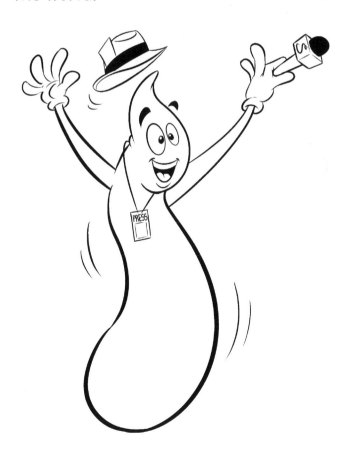

SS - Sausage Shaped

- A Perfect Poo is the shape and size of a big Sausage

- This isn't surprising, Sausage casings used to be pig intestines.

- A good poo retains the shape of the large intestine when it hits the toilet water.

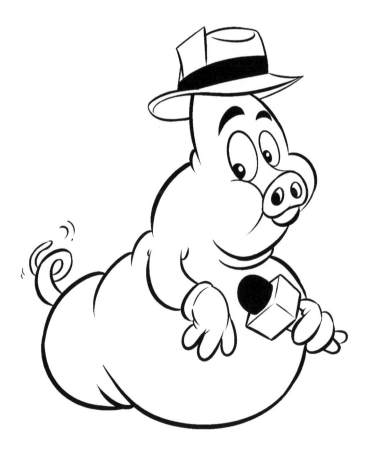

"www.thescooponpoop.ca"

CRAPPY CRAP

C- Concrete

- When the poo comes out hard as rock it is very uncomfortable.

- Sometimes it can be so hard that it becomes impacted in the rectum.

- If you were to poke it with a stick it wouldn't break apart.

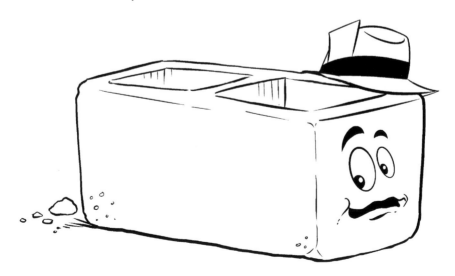

R – Runny

- Sometimes our poo can be more liquid than solid.

- When it is so runny it feels like you are going number 1 instead of number 2, you know things aren't right.

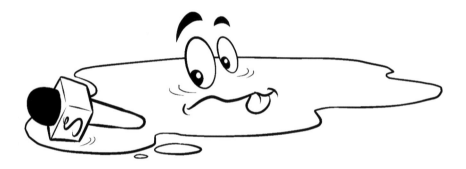

A- Atomic

- This is the explosive bowel movement.

- The one that makes you grateful that you made it to the toilet.

- This kind of release is often accompanied by cramping.

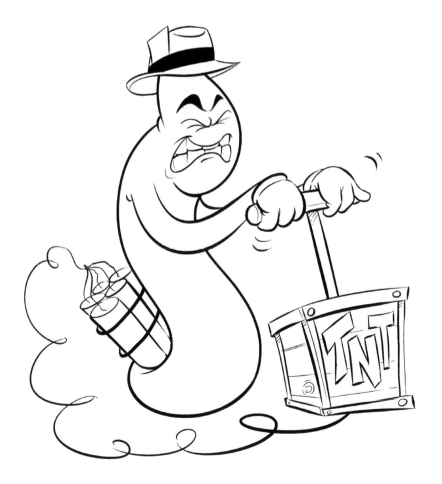

P-Pencil Poop

- This is the stool that's elongated and skinny.

- Sometimes it will curl up in the toilet like a bowl of udon noodles.

- We feel incomplete.

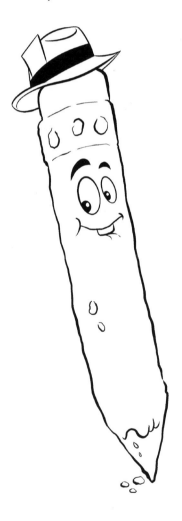

"www.thescooponpoop.ca"

P-Pellet Poop

- Little balls or Pellets similar to Rabbit Feces.

- Completely unsatisfying.

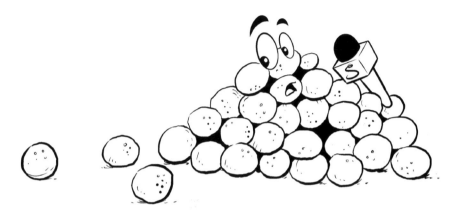

Y-Yucky

- This is like a mud pile.

- Often there is recognizable food products in it.

- It is mushy and thick, a blob

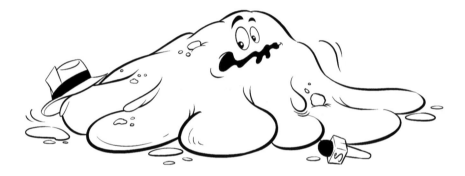

"www.thescooponpoop.ca"

Poo Pondering Questions

What you consume, how you move, how you deal

When pondering your poo ask yourself what did you do in the last 14-24 hours? Whatever you did produced that poo. Remember you are making your poo. What did you do that produced this poo? You are simply observing the truth of cause and effect a Universal Law.

Specifically, what behaviours are we concerned with? We take food, water, light, and oxygen, we stir them with exercise, and bake them with rest, and we have a new us the next day.

There are 3 main behaviors that impact the poo manufacturing process.

1. What you consume.

2. How much you move.

3. How well you manage your bodies physical response to stress.

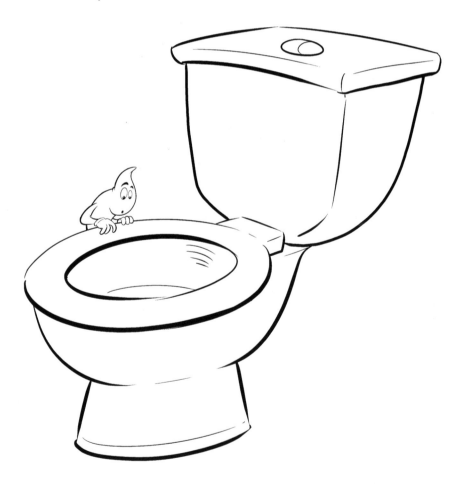

"www.thescooponpoop.ca"

What did I consume in the last 24 hours?

Whatever went in, transformed and came out. These are the ingredients to poo

Whenever looking at how a finished product turned out, we want to consider the ingredients. When it comes to poo, our ingredients are what we consumed.

Consumption includes all liquids and solids ie:

- Water & Herbal Teas

- Veggies and Fruit

- Beans and Grains

- Face Foods (any food that came from something with a face)

- Processed Foods

- Vitamins and Minerals

- Medication

Of the items we consume, the major ingredients that we are concerned with are the four ingredients that make up a good poo. We compare the results of the poop to what we consumed in relationship to those ingredients. The appropriate balance of those ingredients is our goal; that, is what we are figuring out.

We will read a number of different guidelines about proper food, what we want to do is notice the affect on our poo and adjust accordingly. The only person who can be our nutritionist is our-selves; after all, the only person who looks at your poo is you (I hope).

The Ingredients to a Perfect Poop

Water

Ingredient number 1 is water. Pure, clean, an example of the beauty of the exchange between earth and air, water is an essential element. It comes from lakes and rivers, and vegetables, and fruits. We know in our gut that damage to the water is damage to the very life blood of Mother Nature and the life blood of us. On a slightly more mechanical level it is important to understand how water interacts in the body as it travels through the lower intestine.

The small intestine dumps this greenish, oatmeal like sludge called chyme into the large intestine. This chyme is partially digested food and water combined with bile and enzymes. The large intestine grabs the chyme through a process called persistalsis action. The large intestine, or colon, or bowel, is five feet long. The beginning of the bowel, where the colon meets the small intestine is the Cecum. This is where our appendix rests. The peristalsis action absorbs the water back into the body. It travels to the liver for filtering and is then processed through the system, rehydrating the body. It is another example of the awe inspiring perfection of the body. We have this natural defense mechanism which preserves our water.

When the colon shuts down completely our poo is actually chyme or diarrhea. The water and nutrients have not been extracted. The colon is not able to do its' job and we become dehydrated and malnourished.

Now think of the reverse situation. There isn't enough water in the chyme, it gets sucked out one foot into the colon and now we have a dry hard turd that has four more feet to travel. Constipation comes a knocking. Like any organic mixture, it becomes more liquid when we add water. If we want softer poo add more water to the recipe. This is the point where many of my clients will explain that they drink the prescribed eight glasses of water. Let's emphasize that these are just guidelines. The only one who can figure out what works for us is us. Use your poo, add water if it is hard. Reduce it if it is too soft. Everyone uses water differently; some people eliminate it out of their body quickly and need to drink more frequently. However, if we notice a sudden change in your thirst levels over a period of time without any change in behavior or diet, it is wise to see your doctor.

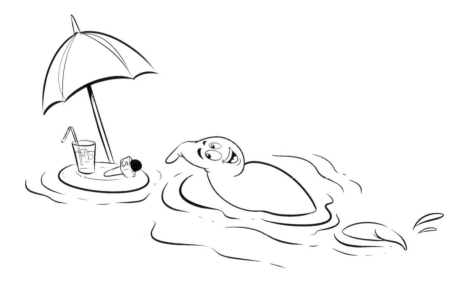

Fiber

The second ingredient is fiber. All Natural Food (except face food) has fiber. If you can pick it or pluck it, it has fiber. Fiber is the stuff that comes out the other end. We don't absorb fiber. It moves through us and out, performing a number of brilliant services in the process.

There are two types of fiber, soluble and insoluble. There is a little of both in all plant based foods but we can identify a plants' primary fiber type by the way it absorbs water.

If it gets bigger when you cook it, it is a soluble fiber. If it doesn't it isn't. Thus, beans and grains are primarily soluble fibers, and nuts, seeds, fruits and vegetables are primarily insoluble.

Both types of fiber are needed to keep a healthy digestive tract. Think of the insoluble fiber as the broom. It sweeps the digestive tract clean. It picks up and scrubs up dead cells, bacteria, bugs, blood, and mucous giving them something to cling to as they move through the entire digestive tract and out the door. It also keeps your transit (the time taken for food to enter and leave the body) at a nice brisk pace, preventing it from slowing down. How does it do that? Both the small and large intestine use peristalsis to move your food through the intestinal track. Think of peristalsis like trying to string an elastic in a waistband. Peristalsis is the physical movement of the fingers as they pinch or pull, however, without a safety pin for the fingers to grasp it is very difficult to string that elastic. Insoluble Fiber is the Safety Pin.

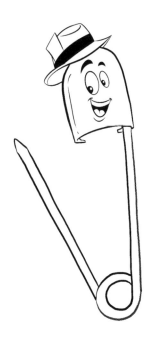

Think of the soluble fiber as the dust pan. It gathers all of the fiber, cells, bacteria, bugs, blood and mucous up into a nice sausage so it is shaped but not hard. Soluble fiber holds on to the water so that the peristalsis of the colon doesn't dry it out too much.

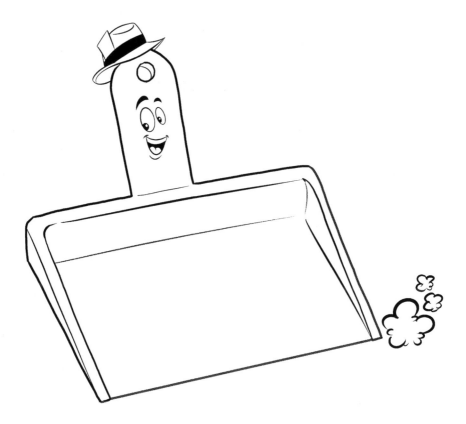

Without both types of fiber your poo will not be very effective. If you don't have any soluble fiber your poo won't form, if you don't have any insoluble fiber your poo will stay in you a long time and you won't clean your digestive tract very well. As with all foods, fiber is affected by processing. Flour based foods are not equivalent to a whole grain or bean. Juicing is not equivalent to the whole fruit or vegetable. So eat lots of fiber, both types, and remember, WHOLE nuts, grains, beans, seeds, vegetables and fruit are your sources

Fat

Ingredient number 3 is fat. Every cell in our body has a membrane that is made with fat. Mothers' milk has a higher percentage of fat than protein. Earlier we talked about fat being an essential macronutrient; however, it also performs a really important function during elimination.

Fat *lubes the tube,* helping the poop slide through the colon easily and pinch off without leaving a sticky mess on the rectum.

If there is no fat in the diet or poor fat in the diet the bowel movement can feel like it's scraping along the walls of the colon as it leaves the rectum. If there is too much fat our poop can end up looking like the blob.

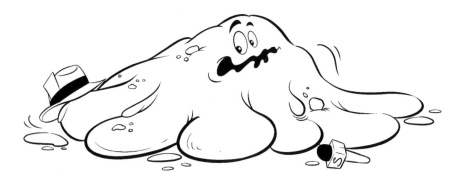

So why has it got such a bad rep? Because, like most things in our lives, fat comes in different guises. We must learn to read through those guises so we can discern the good, the bad, and the ugly.

The Good.

These are poly and mono unsaturated fats, often referred to as Omega-3-6-9. Liquid at room temperature, these fats make cells that are more liquid thus creating a physical body that is more flexible and more responsive. A liquid fat means a liquid you.

Foods that are loaded with these fats are primarily the plant based foods like olives, nuts, seeds, grains, etc. however, fish is also loaded with the Good fats with Salmon and herring vying for supremacy.

The Bad.

These are saturated fats. Hard at room temperature, these fats make your cells hard. Thus, your physical body is harder, and less responsive. Additionally, metabolizing saturated fats produces LDL cholesterol which makes your arteries hard. The harder the fat the harder you are. (and not the good hard). The gristle on a steak is a good example of hard saturated fat.

The UGLY.

These are trans-fats. They do not occur in nature, but are rather the result of processing. Taking those nice liquid fats and heating them so high that the molecular structure of the fat becomes abnormal. Don't kid yourself labelling laws require a list of ingredients, nice mono or poly unsaturated fats may go in, but if it was deep-fried it is still loaded with trans-fat even if the label says 0% trans-fat. Most potato chips are an example of this phenomenon. Read the label and it will say trans-fat free, but test the chip and it will be loaded with trans-fat.

So, it is your choice. Good, Bad or Ugly it will directly affect the kind of body you create and the kind of poo you make.

Good Bacteria

When we are born there are no bacteria in our digestive tract. Up to this point nourishment has been delivered via umbilical cord. We've been using the nutrients, provided by our mothers' blood, to build cells into an actual baby.

Once we are outside the womb we begin to use the digestive tract to access the necessary nutrients. However, there is one little problem. We have no way to absorb those nutrients, because the colonies of bacteria we need aren't set up yet. They still need to move in and multiply. Luckily, it doesn't take long, even without breast feeding (an excellent source of good bacteria) in a few days baby has a nice little colony of these bowel buddies imbedded in the biofilm that lines all of the organs of the digestive tract - and the super pooping begins -.

Good bacteria are the gate keepers, the front line defense of the digestive tract. They perform a major immune function, not allowing undesirables into the body such as bugs, viruses and parasites. Good bacteria are everywhere in the world, but are provided to us primarily through fermented foods.

If you load up on the sauerkraut, or the pickled artichokes, or yogurt, or even a glass of wine (as long as it's just one), you are consuming an excellent source of bowel buddies.

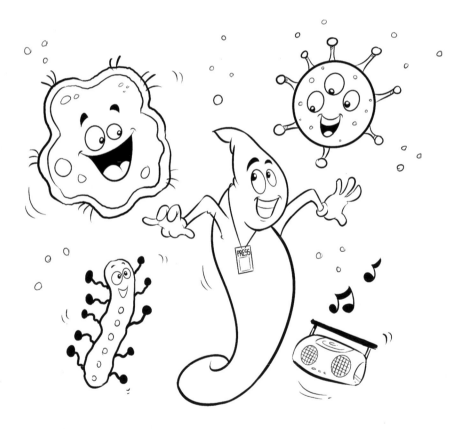

The Ingredients to a Flawed Feces

Processed foods, medications/drugs, supplements

None of the ingredients in small type above should be labeled as bad or good. The reason they are included in this is because their use/misuse are the most common cause of consumption related bowel dysfunction.

The Problems with Processed

Processed food for our purposes will be defined as any food that has been modified by humans. This processing can range from something as simple as peeling, chopping and combining several ingredients into a fruit salad, to stripping, grinding, & bleaching wheat to produce white flour. For our purposes the best guideline is the more processed the food the poorer the poo. This seems like a pretty big generalization, but bare with me as I explain.

Natural food, for the purposes of this book, is what we can eat with little or no tools or processes. This will be food that is recognizable when we look at it such as an apple, a cherry, spinach, a mushroom, a pumpkin seed, a hot pepper, absolutely nothing has been done to it and when we look at it we recognize it for the 1 single food item it is and we can just eat it. It comes with the enzymes that our body needs to break that food down into absorbable nutrients, and send the left over fiber to form a good poop.

Then there is food that is stripped, or soaked, or, boiled, or deboned but still recognizable, which means we can identify its source, such as a filet of chicken, a boiled kidney bean, the meat inside the walnut, a bowl of vegetable chili, because we have to process it a little before we can eat it. Although the enzymes are not as plentiful in the food, our body can still break it down. The general enzymes that our pancreas produces, the bile that the liver produces and the hydrochloric acid that our stomach produces will work on this gently prepared food and then the good bacteria in our digestive track will be able to break it into absorbable nutrients and send the leftovers on to form a good poop. For our purposes we will call this food Healthy Food.

New Food is food we can't identify completely. I cannot look at a piece of bread and tell you what grain was used to make it, thus, bread, pasta and all of the made, simple, white foods like that, are a new food. Most cereals or anything made from flour is a new food. Brownies are a new food, show me a brownie tree, please, I beg you, show me a brownie tree. Most new food has no live enzymes and is re-structured at a molecular level into food our body doesn't know what to do with and thus nutrient absorption is limited and what goes out contains more of what came in. In addition, when the colon tries to form a poop from the leftovers of new food it can be challenged in a myriad of ways.

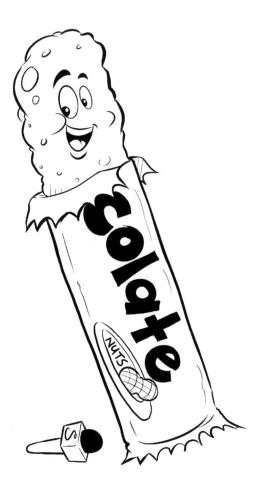

Although a lot of new food is dead food as well, it is important to explain the difference so we can better determine if what was on our plate could be the reason our bowels aren't working. Natural food is loaded with enzymes and bacteria to better help us absorb and eliminate it, dead food has none. Dead food is also often loaded with chemicals, dyes, and extracted single molecule sugars that our body has absolutely no clue how to process. It will often trigger an immune reaction in the digestive tract, causing inflammation and irritation and in turn gas and bloating, because our body doesn't think it is food, thus forming a proper poop is extremely unlikely.

Medications/Drugs

Remember that when we are discussing medications and drugs, we are keeping the conversation within the context of what it does to our poo. We're not interested in moral or ethical choices, nor are we interested in playing the role of doctor. The simple truth is that anything that goes in to the digestive tract will affect the structure of its output. In other words, medications/drugs always impact the way our poo is formed. The good news is that if we know how a particular medication may affect the way we absorb and eliminate, we may be able to counter measure the impact.

There are certain medications, in particular, pain relievers that are notorious for causing constipation. If you are taking such a medication, you will want to compensate with behaviors that soften/moisten your poop and stimulate your transit. There are many different types of antibiotics that we may take to kill bad bacteria that are making us ill, unfortunately, many of them also destroy the good bacteria, our bowel buddies, the ones that help us absorb nutrients and form good poops. Compensating with foods that generate a lot of good bacteria will help negate that negative impact.

The point; is that medication does affect the way bowels form. Whatever drugs or medications we are taking must be allowed for when we are pondering our poo.

Supplements

For our purposes supplements are any processed product which supports the production of or adds essential micronutrients to our body in measurable amounts. For instance, multi-vitamins, protein powder, fish oil, etc. Remember the rule about what goes in comes out? The same is true for supplements and differing amounts of them can really throw off the natural rhythm of the digestive track including such faithfuls as Vitamin C, Magnesium, Iron just to name a few.

If you have inadvertently taken a bit too much Vitamin C or Magnesium, you could well find yourself making an atomic poop or one quite runny. If you have taken too much Iron your bowel movements may put on the brakes so dramatically that you start feeling like you've voluntarily wrapped your abdomen in concrete.

Whatever the supplement, it will impact the formation of the bowel. Good or bad, our poo is an effect of the supplement cause.

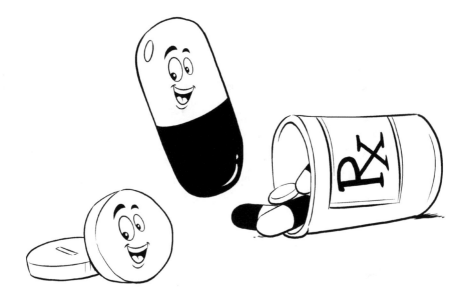

"www.thescooponpoop.ca"

If We Don't Move Our Bowels Don't Move

Movement stimulates the lymphatic system which moves cellular debris out the door.

The large intestine performs a muscular behavior called peristalsis. This muscle is within the walls of the entire tube of the colon and it squeezes and undulates, very much like the movement of an earthworm or a snake.

When we sit for periods of time or fail to stimulate the muscles in our legs, back and abdominals for some reason, our bodies become stiff and our mobility becomes impaired.

The same is true for our bowels. It is a muscle, and like any muscle **if you don't use it you lose it.**

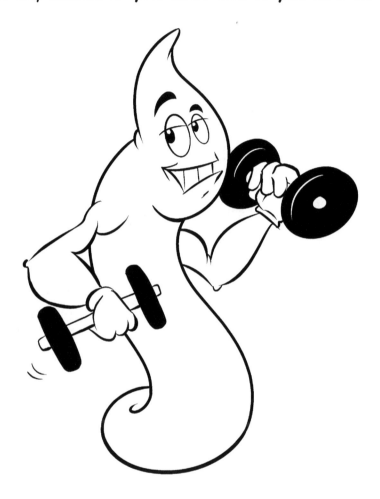

When we don't stimulate our abdominals we can become constipated. Often the people who are the most constipated are those who have jobs that keep them in a sitting position for long periods of time, such as: police officers on stakeout, truckers, office workers etc.

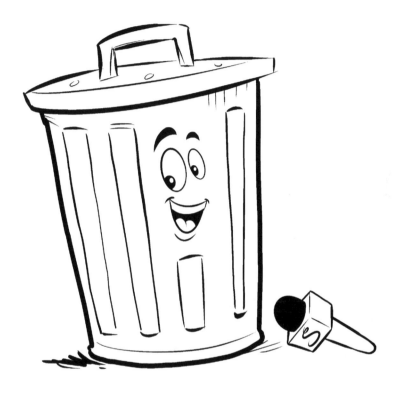

There is an entire system in the physical body known as the lymphatic system. Most of us have heard of the lymph nodes, but we're not really sure what they do. The appendix is a lymph node, the tonsils are lymph nodes and there are a myriad of lymph nodes throughout the body with the largest group being under the arms and in the groin. The lymph nodes produce lymphatic fluid which runs through the body gathering up all the old and dead blood cells, antibodies, and the products of cellular decay and then flushes those things out through our poop. It is our drainage system, and we stimulate it with movement. If we don't move we don't stimulate that system and all those old dead cells have no way to pump out of the body through the colon. Thus once again, we aren't taking out the garbage.

Exercise has a profound effect on good body development and thus proper bowel function.

If you are constipated you may find that regular movement through exercise will alleviate the condition. Running, walking, swimming, dancing, and cycling are all excellent for bowel functioning and help facilitate regularity.

Our bowels are affected by physical activity or non-activity so we can experience constipation with non-activity and even sometimes an over-active bowel when we are over-active as some long-distance runners can attest.

How, much movement have we gotten in the last 12 -24 hours and what is our poop like in relationship to that answer?

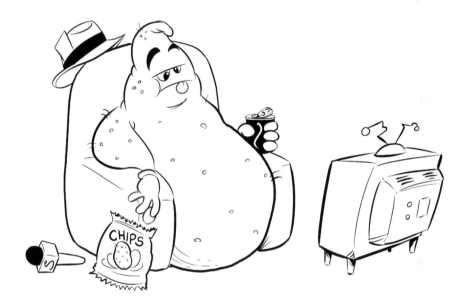

Stress Management

I Think Therefore I Poo

Our emotions have a tremendous impact on the proper (or improper) functioning of our bowels. When we feel good our poo is good, when we feel bad, our poo is bad. There is something called *The Brain Gut Axis* that relates the central nervous system (the brain) with the intestines. Think about your life and times when your bowel functioning has been impacted by your emotions. Perhaps you got nervous before a public speaking engagement and had the runs, or maybe when you get angry you get constipated.

It is what we are thinking that generates our emotions or even more specifically what we believe about what we are thinking. I think and thus I end up feeling. Emotions physically change the way the body works by triggering the release of endorphins, hormones, adrenaline and numerous other chemical substances.

If I **think** I'm in danger, I'll **feel** scared and my body will express that **emotion** (energy in motion) by performing a slew of functions such as;

- Vascular constriction of the core to slow or stop the processes of digestion, absorption, and elimination. The digestive system takes up a tremendous amount of energy to run. When we are in danger, or fleeing for our lives, we need that energy to run, fight, and think, so our beautiful bodies redirect our energy to those functions necessary and elimination is slowed but not stopped. When we are frozen in terror our bowels can lose their muscular control completely and we literally poop our pants.

"www.thescooponpoop.ca"

- Adrenaline and the hormone cortisol flood our blood streams and our senses will go on high alert. We will be in a state of high readiness. We may be able to hear our own heartbeats.

- Our breath becomes shallow and high in the chest. Taking quick little breaths.

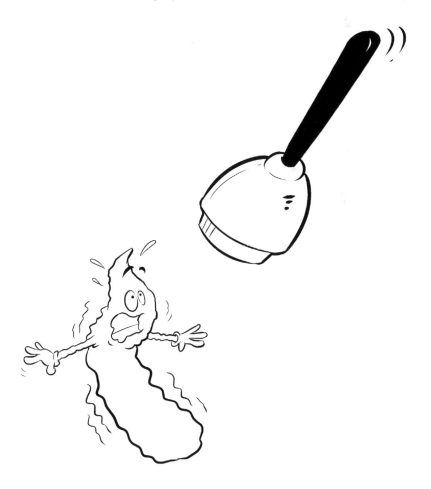

When we are laughing, or happy, we will experience physical changes such as;

- Endorphins flood our blood stream including serotonin, the feel good neurotransmitter. This endorphins improve the way the body processes a number of functions especially in the Brain Gut Axis. Serotonin is used in the gut to digest food and thus create a good poo.

- Clenching of the muscles in the abdominals.

- Deep breathes sometimes to the point of gasping.

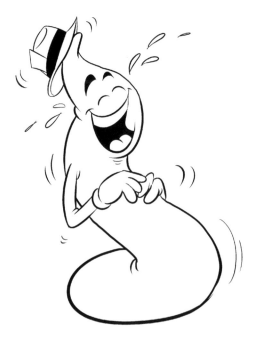

"www.thescooponpoop.ca"

Clearly our body changes with the feelings we experience. Emotions impact the way the body works and the way we build ourselves. Right down to a cellular level. How effective we are at making a good body is directly related to the emotions we generate when we are making it (which is all the time). When you made a good you, you made a good poo. The emotions that we experience throughout the day will have a huge impact on the bowel movements our body forms.

Stress acts just like danger in the body. Our body, in a state of stress, is in the same physiological condition as when it's in danger. When we are stressed, we are running for our lives and we just don't know it. Thus, stress can shut our bowels down. When we don't use it we lose it, so long term stress can cause bowel dysfunction. Because the brain and the bowels are so closely related, it makes sense that the effects of stress can be witnessed in our bowel movements. They are governed by many of the same processes and therefore are interconnected. IBS (irritable bowel syndrome) has been thought to be caused by a dysfunction between the brain and the gut. This means that there is likely a strong connection between the way that we digest food under stress and the bowel movements that we experience. Stress can cause a disruption in the digestion of food, acid reflux and heartburn, all of which can affect proper bowel functioning.

Take the time to reduce the amount of stress you experience in our life and we will notice that our whole body feels better, relaxes and functions better as a result. When thinking about your emotional life and your bowel function, ask yourself; how well am I managing stress in my life? Are you even aware when you are stressed? Most people have physiological indicators that they are stressing. Some of us experience migraines or headaches, others sweat, pace, clench their jaw, have difficulty breathing, get easily irritated, stop eating or overeat, get diarrhea, bite their fingernails, feel nauseous, and many others. Knowing how our body reacts to stress will help us identify it when it occurs. These are our personal indicators, our stress alarms.

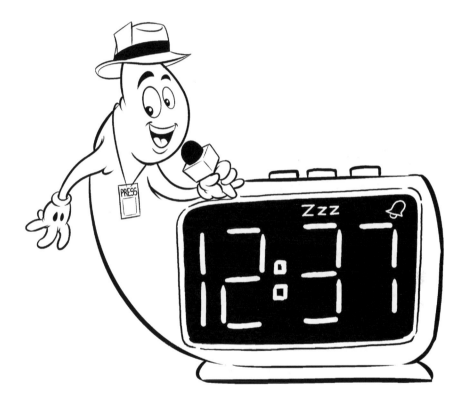

Do you have tactics for transforming your negative stress into emotions that heal and energize your body and thus your poo? The best tactics are those that you can easily, inexpensively, and immediately fit into your lifestyle.

There are 3 behaviors that will stop the stress reaction in the body right in the moment. These behaviors work because they are telling the body that we are ok. These are behaviors that you would never exhibit when you are running for your life, so within a minute of doing any of the following 3 things your body will immediately cease stressing.

Breathe

When we are stressing out, our body moves to a shallow breath from the chest. By consciously changing our breathing pattern to slow and steady from the diaphragm, we are telling our bodies everything is ok. I wouldn't be breathing like a sleeping baby if I had anything to worry about. I'm safe.

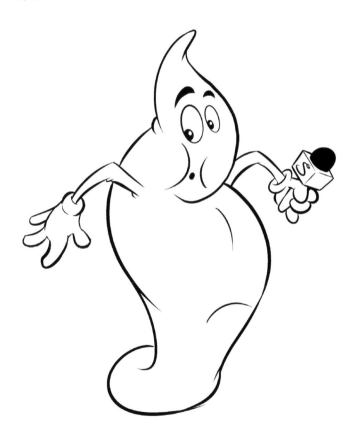

Laugh

We wouldn't laugh if we were running for our life, so as soon as we start laughing we tell our body we are safe. Laughter releases a slew of lovely healthy endorphins, which are a neurotransmitter that tells us are body how to respond in a healthy, cell building, life giving manner. The phrase "Laughter is the Best Medicine", is completely accurate. So a good laugh, even a fake laugh, will start to release the stress reaction. Laughter yoga, is a new type of yoga or meditation, that actually practices forced laughter, it changes breathing, changes chemistry and has an alchemic effect on your body, completely erasing the stress response.

Singing

Certainly no one ever sings or hums when they are running for their life. Choose a few tunes that are uplifting and or soothing and next time you are stewing about a problem as you drive the car. Stop and sing or hum the song instead for at least 2 minutes. You will not be able to retain the stress reaction and you will likely change to a much more pleasant frame of mind.

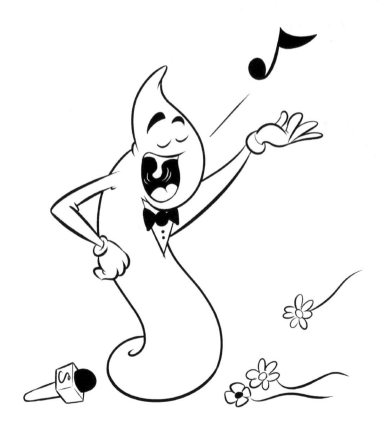

Meditation

Meditation allows us the time and space to focus on our breathing, and clear our mind of all of the mental clutter, stressful thoughts, and pressure of the day. Meditating for even 15 or 20 minutes a day can have a profound effect on our wellbeing and will impact our entire day in a positive way. We will react differently to stress, our body will feel and act better and be more effective, and of course our bowel movements will be more fulfilling and normal than they are when our body is experiencing the physical symptoms of stress.

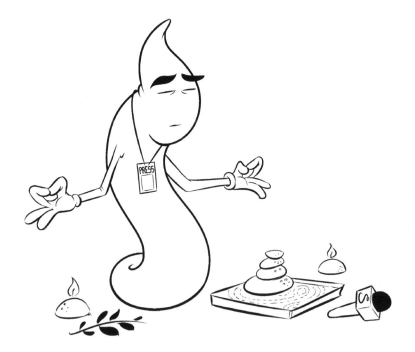

Balanced Diet

We've spoken a great deal about food, but in addition to helping us digest our food properly and facilitating the perfect poo, a balanced diet aids in the management of stress. When we eat the food that our body likes and processes well, everything functions better and we are able to get through the day without feeling tired, depressed or sluggish. Good food revitalizes us and gives us energy. We feel lighter and brighter when we eat whole, organic healthy foods that our body can absorb and digest.

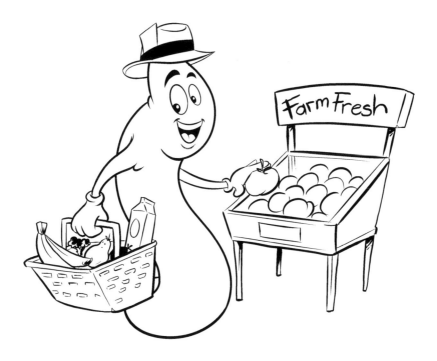

Journaling

Another fantastic means of managing stress is daily journaling. Simply writing down our feelings and getting them down onto the page greatly assists you with emotional blockages. When we don't express how we feel to anyone, we experience a lot of inner stress and turmoil that can affect us in a number of ways. Journaling allows us to sort through our feelings and create a healthy sense of well being, by allowing us to process and work through our stressors without even speaking to anybody. Nobody ever has to see our journal, most people prefer to lock it up or hide it from prying eyes. If we are the only one reading it, we will be much more honest with ourself and in our writing.

Dear Diary...

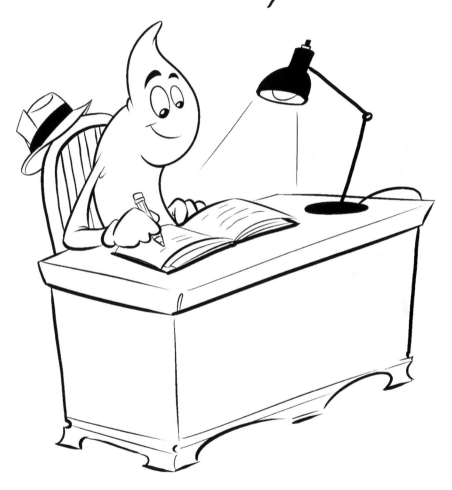

Poo Pondering Conclusions

Whatever you consume, how you move,
and your stress levels create whatever
is smiling back at you from the bowl

Every time we sit down on the toilet to go number two we take that time to ponder our poo. Is it PEERLESS or CRAPPY?

What did we consume in the last 14 to 24 hours? Because what's in the bowl is made up of that.

How much movement did we get? Because what's in the bowl was stirred by that.

How well did we handle our stress? Because what's in the bowl was baked by that.

When you correlate the results of your pondering you can figure out what works for you and now you know the scoop on poop and how to make a perfect poo.

When Bowels Go Bad

What to do when you have chronic Constipation/Diarrhea/bloating and the doctors say there is nothing wrong.

Most people will suffer from bouts of constipation, or diarrhea at least a few times in their life. These bouts can be caused from a myriad of different problems such as bad bacteria, or bugs, food that's taken a turn, over indulgence, a virus etc.

However, there are a slew of people who suffer from bowel disruption on a chronic basis. They've been to the doctors, and had the tests. All the genetic causes have been eliminated. They haven't been able to identify any diseases that could be causing the problem. All allergies and food sensitivities have been accounted for, and yet they suffer on an ongoing and frequent basis. These poor souls often get lumped into a growing category, called irritable bowel syndrome or IBS. Sound familiar? If it does, take heart. If you apply the principles outlined in this book, using your poo to self actualize your behavior, you will likely be able to change the condition you find yourself in. As an added bonus, there is a process that you can undergo, which will jump start this change and help get your colon back into toned working condition.

Get a series of colonics and apply the principles in this book and you will be on your way to making a PERFECT POO!!

Colon Hydrotherapy

Colonics perform 3 major roles; exercising and cleaning the colon, and hydrating the body.

Colon Hydrotherapy or Colonics is the gentle introduction of water into the bowel triggering the client to poop, over and over again. Effectively making you poo more than you ever have before. It is a marathon pooing session. Colonics perform 3 major roles; exercising and cleaning the colon, and hydrating the body.

Exercising

The colons' main functions are to re-absorb nutrients and water into our bodies and eliminate toxic waste. Our bowel movements are what make this happen, but when the machine isn't a well-oiled one, we can face some serious problems including the slowing of the bowel. When the bowel gets impacted we begin to experience problems like haemorrhoids, constipation, or more serious things like colon cancer. There are dozens of complications and conditions that can arise from the presence of a movement challenged colon.

In fact bowel dysfunction is very common these days due to the poor nature of the Western diet, our sedentary life style and our egregious stress management skills. When you tack on tea, coffee, alcohol, and a lack of water to that – it's not looking good.

Perhaps we have decided to change our ways, but we still have a sad immobile bowel that doesn't have a clue when to poo. This is where colon hydrotherapy comes in. Having colon hydrotherapy is like taking the colon to the gym. It is a work out for the colon. The colon performs a muscular behaviour called peristalsis, when the muscle loses its' tone its' out of shape. Colonics are the introduction of water into the bowel to trigger the behaviour of the bowel. It's like putting the colon on a treadmill, improving the function of the bowel.

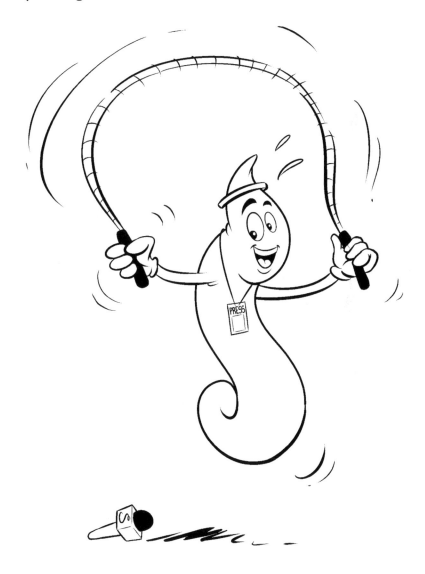

Cleansing

Colonics are an important part of detoxification. It's not just the food we eat that creates toxins in the body, it is also pharmaceutical products, the air we breathe, and even the products we use. All of these things go through our bodies and can create toxemia.

Toxins in the bio-film of the bowel create more than just problems in the bowels. They can cause a whole host of diseases, conditions and even death. Intestinal toxicity is a profound and common problem in Western Society. When the toxins in your body have built up to such a point that you are demonstrating signs of dysfunction, then we don't want to wait for good bacteria to do its job. Colon Hydrotherapy will cleanse the old, and the triggering of the behaviour of the colon will cause any hard old bio-film to be broken up and eliminated, making room for fresh healthy colonies of bacteria.

If you are eating poorly, stressed out, not sleeping or exercising and not drinking enough water, a cleanse will benefit you greatly by helping you clear out toxicity from your body. Good bacteria are built up through proper lifestyle choices, healthy eating and regiments, but sometimes we have to clear out the remnants of poor decisions of our past to restore our intestinal health. It is true that healthy eating and lifestyle will help your body naturally clear itself of chemicals, toxins and harmful bacteria, but it takes time to do this, and unless you are eating live perfectly every day all day and have been doing so for the past several years, then you will benefit greatly from a gentle and safe colon cleanse.

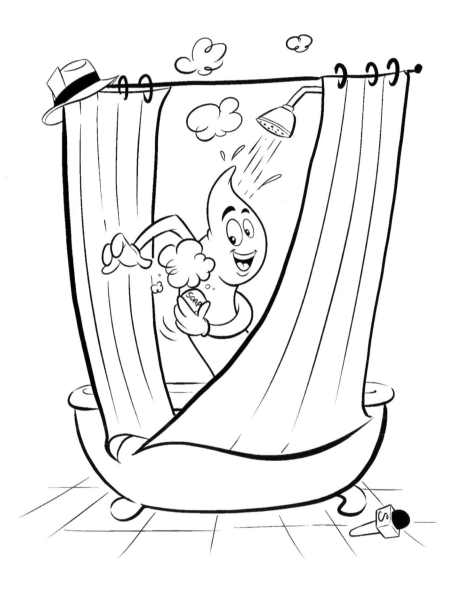

"www.thescooponpoop.ca"

Hydrating

When the small intestine drops the chyme into the colon, the colon grabs this thick liquid and using peristalsis extracts the water. The water gets carried to the liver where it gets cleaned and is used to hydrate the body. Colon Hydrotherapy introduces super filtered water into the colon and triggers peristalsis, effectively causing some of that pure water to flush up to the liver. Hydrating the body and giving the liver a nice bath.

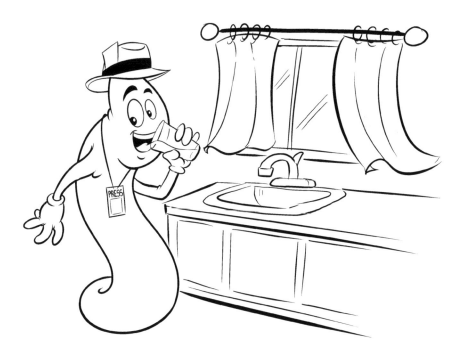

Choosing What Colonic is Right for You

Open or closed colonics pros or cons

There are 2 types of colonics, open or closed. Both colonics are effective, both colonics work equally well, however they are different from a process perspective, so it is wise to consider this when looking for a colonics provider. Open colonics differ from closed colonics on the following points.

Feature	Closed	Open
Rectal Tubes	Large rectal tube to accommodate water delivery and pipe the feces to the sewage system	Tiny tube since it delivers water only.

Table	Flat examination Table	Lounging Toilet
Privacy	The therapist must stay in the room to switch between water input and client output, and to hold the rectal tube in place	Therapist can leave the room, since client just poos around the tiny tube and down into the toilet.
You can Pee	No	Yes
Finishing	Client must move quickly to a toilet and sit there until they are finished	Client can finish on the system.

At Elemental Therapies, this authors business, we use the open colon hydrotherapy system "The Angel of Water" TM for our colonic services. If you are interested in finding out more about colonics you can go to our website at www.elementaltherapies.ca or email info@elementaltherapies.ca.

Printed in the United States
By Bookmasters